Kyaw Naing Win
Rizal Sablee

Noise Induce Hearing Loss

Kyaw Naing Win
Rizal Sablee

Noise Induce Hearing Loss

LAP LAMBERT Academic Publishing

Impressum / Imprint

Bibliografische Information der Deutschen Nationalbibliothek: Die Deutsche Nationalbibliothek verzeichnet diese Publikation in der Deutschen Nationalbibliografie; detaillierte bibliografische Daten sind im Internet über http://dnb.d-nb.de abrufbar.

Alle in diesem Buch genannten Marken und Produktnamen unterliegen warenzeichen-, marken- oder patentrechtlichem Schutz bzw. sind Warenzeichen oder eingetragene Warenzeichen der jeweiligen Inhaber. Die Wiedergabe von Marken, Produktnamen, Gebrauchsnamen, Handelsnamen, Warenbezeichnungen u.s.w. in diesem Werk berechtigt auch ohne besondere Kennzeichnung nicht zu der Annahme, dass solche Namen im Sinne der Warenzeichen- und Markenschutzgesetzgebung als frei zu betrachten wären und daher von jedermann benutzt werden dürften.

Bibliographic information published by the Deutsche Nationalbibliothek: The Deutsche Nationalbibliothek lists this publication in the Deutsche Nationalbibliografie; detailed bibliographic data are available in the Internet at http://dnb.d-nb.de.

Any brand names and product names mentioned in this book are subject to trademark, brand or patent protection and are trademarks or registered trademarks of their respective holders. The use of brand names, product names, common names, trade names, product descriptions etc. even without a particular marking in this work is in no way to be construed to mean that such names may be regarded as unrestricted in respect of trademark and brand protection legislation and could thus be used by anyone.

Coverbild / Cover image: www.ingimage.com

Verlag / Publisher:
LAP LAMBERT Academic Publishing
ist ein Imprint der / is a trademark of
OmniScriptum GmbH & Co. KG
Heinrich-Böcking-Str. 6-8, 66121 Saarbrücken, Deutschland / Germany
Email: info@lap-publishing.com

Herstellung: siehe letzte Seite /
Printed at: see last page
ISBN: 978-3-659-80054-2

Noise Induced Hearing Loss

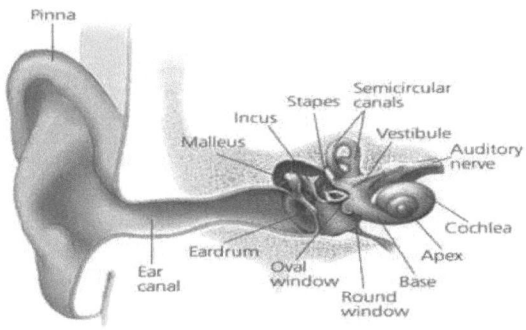

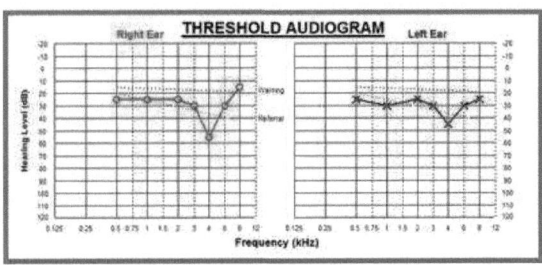

Contents

Epidemiology

Excessive noise is fast becoming a global occupational health hazard and is associated with considerable physiological and social effects. It is estimated that worldwide, occupational noise has been a source of disabling hearing loss in approximately 16% of adults with effects seen to be higher in males and in developing countries (Nelson DI, et al, 2005). The World Health Organization currently estimates that 250 million people worldwide have disabling hearing loss of moderate to profound severity. Adult-onset hearing loss ranks fifteenth in the list of leading causes of Global Burden of Disease (GBD), and second in the list of leading causes of Years Lived with a Disability (YLD) (WHO, 2015). In United State, 10% of adult hearing loss is due to occupational exposure and it is the most significant preventable cause of hearing loss (Dobie, 2007). The Norwegian Labour Inspectorate in 2006 reported 3392 cases of work related diseases, of which 59% were due to noise-induced hearing loss (NIHL) (Samant Y, et al, 2008). Noise induced hearing loss (NIHL) is most prevalent, but is also the most preventable occupational disease in the majority of developing Asian Countries. The highest proportion of adult-onset hearing loss in the world results from noise exposure in Asian Countries. This is partly due to the developing economies of these countries where there are limitations in health services and preventative programmes. One other major factor is the lack of awareness of NIHL amongst employers and employees (Fuente A and Hickson L, 2011). In Australia, it were estimated that occupational noise accounted for 10% of adult-onset hearing loss. Between 2002 to 2007, 16500 accepted worker compensation claims in Australia was for deafness due to noise exposure. 65% of these claims are made up of the manufacturing, construction and transport industries (Steve C, et al, 2010). In Brazil, metal working accounted for around 16% of all NIHL cases. Similar numbers have been found for coal mine workers in the US. Other jobs that are of high risk of acquiring NIHL include those in the aviation industry, uniform personnel (army, police, and firefighters), heavy goods vehicle drivers and professional divers (Azizi MH, 2010). Police officers are potentially exposed to multiple sources of noise, including vehicle horns, gunfire, barking from police dog and traffic noise (Mc Combe AW, et al, 1995). Specifically for police motorcyclists, the noise exposure can range from 63 to 90 dBA, and up to 105 dBA in open road (Ross BC, 1989).

Physics of Sound

Noise is defined as 'unwanted sound', and is produced by the phenomenon of fluctuations in atmospheric pressure. Sound is created by oscillations/pressure variation in an elastic medium and confined to air. Sound travels in the form of longitudinal waves, which involves compressions and rarefractions within the air.

However, the topic of sound can be very much subjective i.e. one person's sound can be another's noise. Noise being a source of serious health effect, has only been recognised due to the development of modern times, with humans being increasingly reliant on the use of modern transportation and technology. With the recent development of industrialization, industrial noise has significant contributory factor for noise induced hearing loss.

Simplified, sound waves are characterised by:

Wavelength

The distance a wave travels in one cycle.

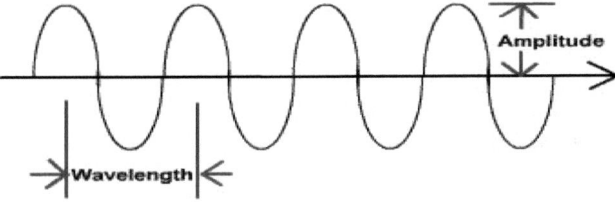

Frequency

The number of cycles per second and it is measured in Hz (1 Hz is 1 cycle per second). Audible frequency range for a healthy young listener is 20-20000 Hz. Sensitivity to higher frequencies decrease with age and noise exposure.

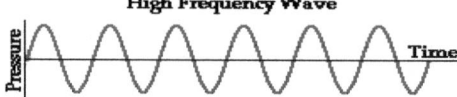

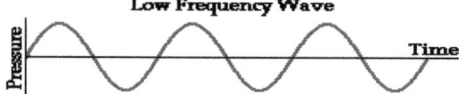

Period

The time taken for one cycle to pass a fixed point (Period = 1/frequency). Speed of sound = 343m/s @20°C and 1 atmospheric pressure.

Sound pressure levels

This refers to the measure by which air vibrations make up sound. A healthy human ear is able to detect a wide range of sound pressure levels, from 10 to 102 pascal (Pa). Due to this wide range, an algorithmic scale is used, converting to the internationally known units of decibels (dBA). The minimum acoustic pressure that is audible is 20×10^{-6} Pa and occurs at 4000 Hz. On the other end of the scale, pain is caused by sounds pressures in the order of 60pa.

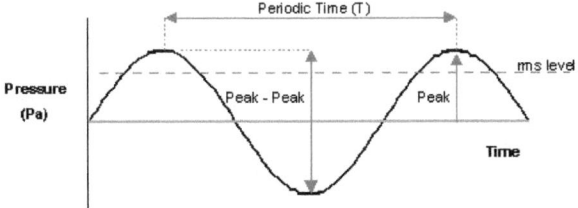

Frequency Weighting

Not all frequencies are relevant to our daily lives. As such, a frequency weighting network has been developed with the aim of providing a much simpler approach by considering the weighting of the important frequencies collectively into a single number rating. The most commonly used is the A-weighting system, whereby low frequencies are less weighted than mid – higher frequency sounds (Hansen CH, 1995).

Types of Noise

Noise is an unwanted, undesirable and sometimes damaging sound. It can be classified as continuous or steady state, fluctuating, intermittent and impulsive noise.

Steady or continuous noise is a sound those with noise with negligibly small fluctuations of sound pressure level within the period of observation which is generally less than 3 dBA. Examples of these noises include electrical generators, printing machine and waving machine.

Fluctuating noise is a sound when the pressure levels shift significantly during the period of observation. The intensity of noise is usually varies more than 3dBA.

Intermittent noise is sound whose intensity drops to the ambient level several times, e.g; noise cause by chain saw to cut logs.

Impulsive noise is a sound with a sudden change of intensity of at least 40 dBA with short duration generally less than 0.5 second e.g; noise from fire arm (Hansen CH, 1995).

Hearing Mechanism

Hearing, like vision, is one of human's most precious senses. It is used in communicating and also as important, used to detect warnings from a distance. As described earlier, sound travels through air via vibrations, and this is picked up by the ear. The function of the ear is to convert these vibrations in physical form into nerve impulses which can then vitally inform the higher parts of the brain. A simple analogy of how the ear functions is by looking at a microphone, whereby the mechanism is similar i.e. converting vibrations into an electrical signal.

Structurally the ear is made up of the outer, middle (both called responsible for sound conduction) and inner parts (responsible for sound transduction).

Outer Ear

The pinna (the outermost part of the outer ear) protrudes from the side of the skull and functions by collecting sound and channelling it into the ear canal. The ear canal (external acoustic meatus) itself is approximately 4cm in length, consisting of hairs, sweat and sebaceous glands which work together to form earwax. The base of the ear canal is where the tympanic membrane lies. The outer layer of this is made from the same skin as that of the ear canal. The whole tympanic membrane is less than $1/10^{th}$ of a mm thick and is connected to the middle ear space.

Middle ear

The middle ear contains three little bones (malleus, incus and stapes) and it is these bones that conduct sound from the tympanic membrane (the outer wall of the middle ear) to the cochlear (inner wall of the middle ear). The structure of the middle ear itself is of an air filled space that is connected to the back of the nose via the Eustachian tube. This tube is bony in nature as it leaves the middle ear but becomes cartilage and muscle as it nears the back of the nose. Those muscles actively open the tubes, allowing pressure in the middle ear and nose to equalise. This is the reason that some people often complain of blocked nose and a sensation of a 'blocked ear' at the same time.

Inner ear

The cochlea is akin to a snail shell due to its appearance being that of two and a half turns which houses the membranous labyrinth and is filled with fluid. Incredibly, this space contains up to 30,000 hair cells which functions by transducing vibration into nervous impulses and around 19000 nerve fibres which carry the signal to and from the brain.

The sound conducting mechanism of the ear has a range of audible sound in the frequency range 16 Hz to 20,000 Hz. Sensitivity is low at the extremes but best between 128Hz up to 4kHz where it then becomes much less sensitive thereafter. It is important to note that the range of maximum sensitivity diminishes with age.

The sound transducing mechanism i.e. the inner ear also analyses the frequency and intensity of sound. Nerve impulses produced by the inner ear are carried from the cochlea to the brain stem via the 8th Cranial Nerve (Hansen CH, 1995).

Pathophysiology of Noise Induced Hearing Loss

Mechanical Process

The various mechanical processes that could cause damage to the hair cells as a result of high intensity noise exposure which includes:

1. Violent fluid motion in the cochlear partition from exposure to loud noise causing tips of stereocilia on the outer hair cell to be removed from the point of insertion with the tectorial

membrane. In addition, the stereocilia may be broken leading to loss of structural integrity.

2. Damage to pillar cell and supporting cell (Deiters's and Hensen's) leading to interfere with local vibration along the organ of Corti.

3. Damage to hair cells either directly by detaching the organ of Corti or tearing of basilar membrane.

4. Rupture of Reissner's membrane with mixing of endolymph and perilymph resulting in damage to the hair cell.

However, the more common sustained, prolonged noise exposure will often cause hair cell damage by metabolic exhaustion as well as glycogen depletion and ischemia induced by changes in cochlear microcirculation will eventually result in cell death via necrosis or apoptosis.

Metabolic Process

The metabolic process that could damage hair cell as a result of noise exposure includes:

1. Overstimulation of outer hair cell, making them requires more energy. Vesiculation and vacuolation in endoplasmic reticulum of the hair cells lead to cell membrane rupture and hair cell loss.

2. Hair cell loss may be due to metabolic exhaustion as a result of disruption of enzyme system.

3. Rises in the intra-cellular calcium level in outer hair cell lead to cytoskeletal breakdown, membrane defects and DNA damage.

4. Reduction in cochlear blood flow which will lead to hair cell loss.

5. Glutamate excitotoxicity will cause swelling and rupturing of auditory afferent nerve fibres.

The region of the organ of Corti is about 8 to 10 mm from basal end which is corresponding to 4 kHz region of the audiogram and uniquely vulnerable to noise which cause typical notch around the 4 kHz region in NIHL. Several theories have been mentioned on why NIHL initially involves surroundings 4 Khz region, and they include:

1. The harmonic amplification theory: The physical structure of ear canal creates a resonance and amplifies frequencies at 2-3 kHz. Hence, although occupational noise is mostly broad band, the energy that is most likely transmitted to the cochlea in the 2-3 kHz regions. Maximum hearing loss usually occurs about one or half an octave above the exposure frequency.

2. The absolute sensitivity theory: The ear is most sensitive in the 4kHz region which is shown in psychoacoustic studies.

3. The biomechanical theory: The energy is being transferred middle ear into the endolymph is greatest as it goes through

the first bend of the cochlea. The hair cells are located at the first bend are those representing approximately 4 kHz.

4. Middle ear muscle contraction: Chronically intense loud sounds will make the middle ear muscle contract and reduced only the transmission of low frequency into the cochlea, as opposed to the acute contraction of the muscles which will block the transmission of sound for all frequencies (Koh D and Takahashi K, 2011).

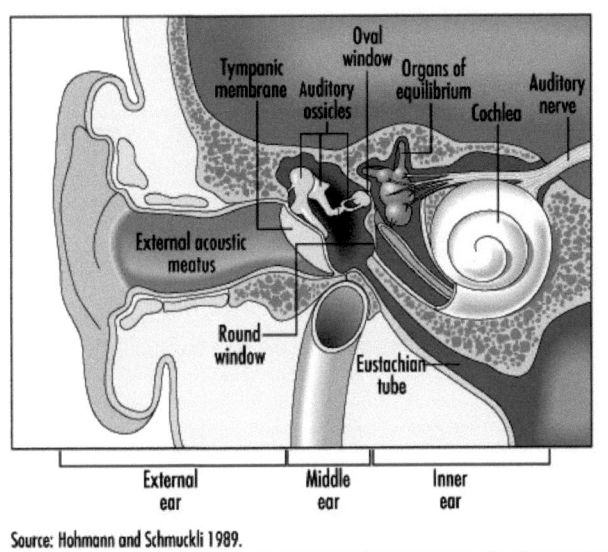

Source: Hohmann and Schmuckli 1989.

Ref: Boillat MC. Chapter 11. Sensory Sytems. ILO encyclopedia. 2015.
http://www.ilocis.org/documents/chpt11e.htm

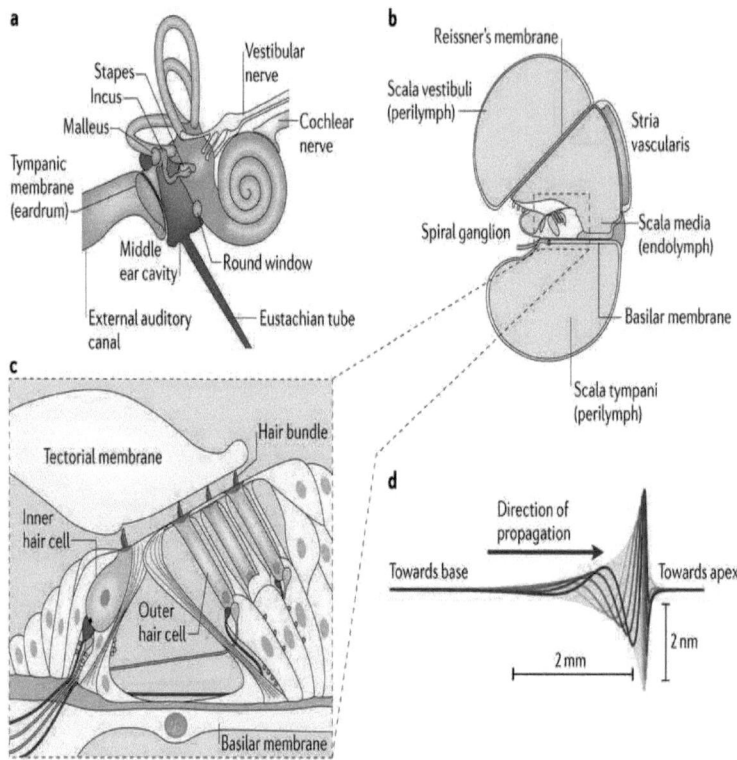

a

Stapes
Incus
Malleus
Tympanic membrane (eardrum)
Vestibular nerve
Cochlear nerve
Middle ear cavity
Round window
External auditory canal
Eustachian tube

b

Reissner's membrane
Scala vestibuli (perilymph)
Stria vascularis
Scala media (endolymph)
Spiral ganglion
Scala media (endolymph)
Basilar membrane
Scala tympani (perilymph)

c

Tectorial membrane
Hair bundle
Inner hair cell
Outer hair cell
Basilar membrane

d

Direction of propagation
Towards base
Towards apex
2 mm
2 nm

Nature Reviews | Neuroscience

14

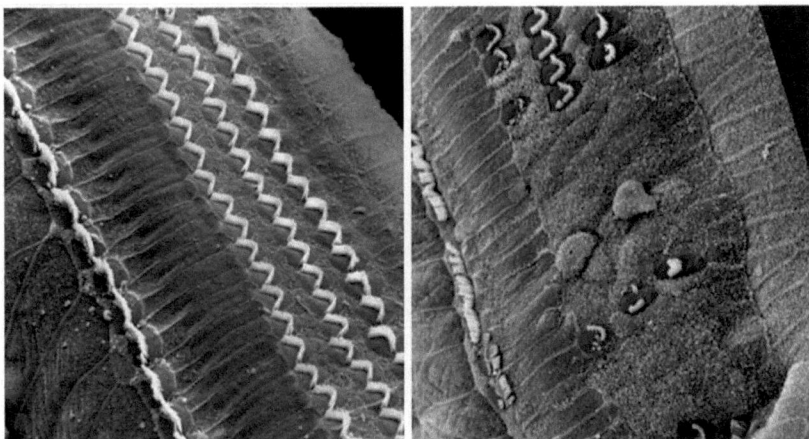

Intact cochlea   Damaged cochlea

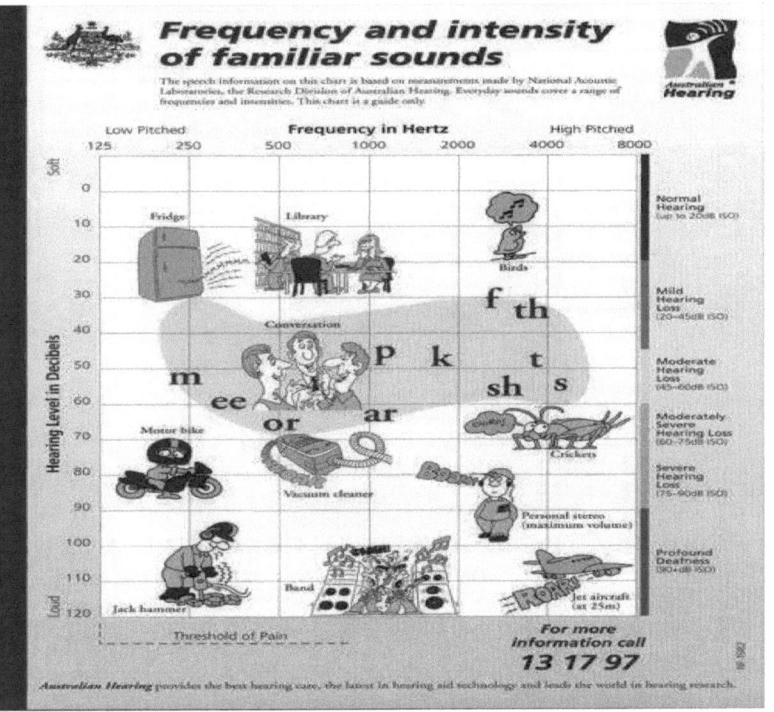

Adverse Health effects of noise

Sound is essential for the satisfaction of everyday life whether it be from children playing in the park, from communication with family and friends, and even music. However, noise pollution can cause significant adverse effects as will be mentioned below.

Noise-induced hearing impairment

This type of impairment is typically defined by the increasing in hearing threshold and is commonly assessed via audiometry. It is the most prevalent irreversible occupational hazard worldwide. For developing countries, both occupational and environmental noises are two of the largest factors contributing to hearing impairment. Studies have shown that noise-induced hearing impairment predominantly occurs at high frequencies (from 3kHz to 6kHz), with the largest effect seen at 4kHz. ISO and WHO have specified that 8 hour exposure times at occupational noise levels below 75dBA should not result in noise-induced hearing impairment. Socially, the main consequence of hearing impairment is the inability to comprehend speech during daily living conditions and this is considered to be a severe handicap. Even 10dBA average hearing impairment over the 2kHz to 4kHz range over both ears is enough to affect the understanding of speech. It has been recommended that to reduce the risk of hearing impairment, 24 hr average noise exposure values of 70dBA and below should be observed. For impulse noise exposures, this should never exceed 140dBA for adults and 120dBA for children.

Sleep Disturbance

This is considered a major environment noise effect. The primary effects of sleep disturbance include:

- Difficulty falling asleep
- Reduction in the proportion of REM-sleep
- Increased blood pressure
- Increased Heart Rate
- Cardiac arrhythmia
- Increase in body movements

Secondary effects are effects felt by the person the following day and these include:

- Reduced perceived sleep quality
- Increased fatigue
- Depressed mood/well-being
- Decreased work performance

It's believed that for a good night's sleep, indoor noise levels should not exceed 45dB more than 10-15 times at night (Vallet & Vernet 1991).

Cardiovascular effects

Studies have shown that noise may possibly a risk factor cardiovascular disease. Workers exposed to high levels of industrial noise for at least 5 yrs have increased blood pressure and are at an increased risk for hypertension and ischaemic heart disease.

Social and Behavioural effects

Noise can produce a number of social and behavioural effects, annoyance particularly in community noise exposure.

Effects of noise on performance

Studies have shown that noise can act as a distracting stimulus. Noise-induced arousal may produce better performance for simple tasks. However, more complex tasks that required high cognitive performances deteriorates noticeably such as having to sustain attention to details or for multitasking duties. Chronic exposure to aircraft noise during early childhood has been shown to impair reading acquisition and reduce motivation.

Guideline values for community noise in specific environment

Specific Environment	Critical Health Effects	LAeq (Average) in dB	Time base (hours)
Indoor dwelling	Speech intelligibility, annoyance daytime & Evening	35	16
Inside bedroom	Sleep disturbance, night time	30	8
Industrial, commercial shopping and traffic areas.	Hearing Impairment	70	24
Ceremonies, festivals and entertainment events (<5 times/year)	Hearing Impairment	100	4
Music through headphones	Hearing Impairment	85	1
Impulse sounds from toys, fireworks and firearms	Hearing Impairment	L Max: 140 (Adults) 120 (Children)	-

Ref: (Birgitta B, et al, 1999)

DECIBEL SCALE (dBA)

- Threshold of pain — 130
- Rock band
- 120 — 747 on take off
- 110
- Jackhammer
- Heavy truck — 100
- Medium truck
- 90
- Passenger car — 80
- Normal conversation at 1 to 2 m
- 70
- Suburban residential neighbourhood — 60
- 50
- 40
- Quiet living room
- Quiet rural setting — 30
- 20 — Whisper
- 10
- 0 — Threshold of hearing

Types of NIHL

Noise-induced hearing loss (NIHL) is sensory neural hearing loss due to exposure to intense impulse or continuous sound. The exposure of noise can be occupational or non-occupational.

There are basically two different types of NIHL

> ➤ *NIHL caused by Acoustic Trauma*

This refers to permanent damage to the cochlear from a single exposure to excessive sound (in most cases a sound impulse) such as explosions, gunfire and firecrackers.

> ➤ *Gradually developing NIHL*

This also refers to permanent damage to the cochlear but from repeated exposures to excessive noises.

Since decibels (dB) are based on a logarithmic scale, every increase of 10dB equates to a doubling of sound intensity. This is important because gradually developing NIHL occurs from both the exposure to sounds intensity and its duration.

Temporary Threshold Shift (TTS)

The outer hair cells which are located in the external canal are most sensitive to ototoxic medication and chemicals. Once they are damaged, it may result in a 40dB increase in hearing threshold. The inner hair cells which are located in cochlea may be damaged by intense acoustic stimuli. Once these cells are damaged, they are not regenerated and so hearing deficits are permanent.

There is a phenomenon called the threshold shift which can be temporary or permanent. These results from increased levels of noise exposure. TTS increases in severity by 6dB for every doubling in intensity of noise exposure. As the name suggests, TTS is entirely reversible but may persist for a few hours after noise exposure ceases. It is important to note however that repeated noise exposures may result in reduced hearing recovery, resulting in permanent threshold shift (PTS) which is due to the degeneration of hair cells (Birgitta B, et al, 1999).

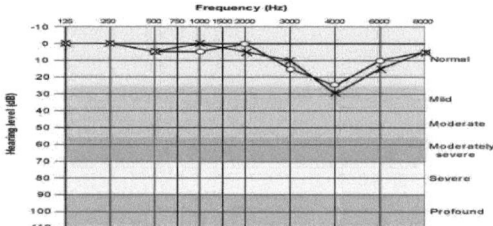

Noise Induced Hearing Loss in the Police Force in Brunei Darussalam

In Brunei Darussalam, all Royal Brunei Police Force (RBPF) personnel are required to undergo shooting practice at least annually or when required. The provision and compulsory use of hearing protection devices such as ear muffs were introduced into the RBPF since 2005. Prior to this, RBPF personnel with exposure to excessive noise, particularly during shooting practices or in job designations such as police motorcyclists or traffic police, did not have any hearing protection at all. The discovery of a number of NIHL among these police personnel led the study team to carry out a survey to estimate the prevalence of NIHL in this working population, as well as study the relationship between NIHL and its associated factors. Further to this, we aimed to assist the RBPF force in the implementation of a hearing conservation program as a control measure in the prevention of NIHL. The introduction of such a program could also be adopted in other work places with excessive noise levels.

The Occupational Health Division (OHD) conducts periodic medical examinations for RBPF personnel at the non-officer level 3-yearly when their job contractual agreement is due for expiry. RBPF personnel who are non-officers hold posts of different ranks such as Police Constable, Lance Corporal, Corporal, Sergeant, Staff Sergeant, and Sergeant Major.

In this study, the medical examinations included obtaining a detailed occupational history, significant past medical history, past and current noise exposure history as well as compliance with usage of hearing protective devices, and physical examination which included body mass index and otoscopic examination for external ear conditions such as ear drum perforation, ear wax impaction or external ear infections. Other tests such as full blood count, fasting blood sugar, fasting cholesterol, liver function tests, renal function tests and urine microscopy as well as audiometry test, were done to complete the medical examination. Audiometry was done at least 16 hours after the last noise exposure to exclude temporary threshold shift (TTS), a condition where there is temporary hearing loss after noise exposure.

Audiometric testing at OHD is conducted using a screening audiometer (model AS 208) manufactured by inter acoustic A/S (Denmark). This is usually carried out by doing air conduction test at frequencies of 500, 1000, 2000, 3000, 4000 & 6000Hz taken for each ear in a closed room environment with minimal ambient noise level of 20 to 25 dBA. Further information obtained by face to face interview with an occupational health nurse at this stage would include any history of hobbies with possible excessive noise exposure such as listening to loud music, singing or karaoke activities, part time work in a noisy environment, recent ear infection, history of head and/or neck injury, exposure to chemicals and ototoxic medications or a family history of hearing loss. Severity of NIHL is based on the World Health Organization (WHO) grading. Hearing within 0 to 25 dBA or less (better ear) is classified as normal hearing, 26 to 40 dBA as mild impairment, 41 to 60 dBA as moderate impairment, 61 to 80 dBA as severe impairment, and over 80 dBA as profound impairment (WHO, 2008). Environmental noise level at the shooting range was not measured due to inaccessibility.

Study Design and Study Population

A cross sectional study was conducted on police personnel at non-officer level employed with the RBPF, who were seen for periodic medical examination at OHD during the period of January 2012 until December 2012. Each subject had to have been in service for at least three years and a maximum of thirty years. Diagnosis of NIHL was based on (i) history of occupational noise exposure, (ii) bilateral hearing loss, (iii) hearing loss of >25 dBA at 4000 Hertz frequency in two consecutive audiograms and (iv) no significant past medical history affecting hearing[11]. Other causes of hearing loss needed to be excluded such as non-occupational noise exposure, ototoxic medications, family history of hearing loss, recent or chronic ear infections, head and neck injury, radiotherapy to the head and neck, and history of mumps. New police recruits during this period were also excluded. Of note, part of the selection criteria to join the RBPF was absence of any hearing impairment. Smoking and alcohol consumption were included as part of the demographic data. In cases where NIHL was diagnosed, the individual was referred to the ENT department at a tertiary hospital for further diagnostic and confirmatory tests.

Data Collection and Statistical Analysis

Collection of data was done by the study team from OHD by reviewing the clinical records. Relevant information was collected from the findings of routine periodic medical examination that police personnel undergo at the OHD. The information was entered into a database for study analysis as well as for the Division's record keeping. Statistical analysis was done using SPSS version 16 for Windows.

Data analysis was done by using Pearson Chi Square tests and risk estimation by Odds Ratio. It was found that there was a significant association between NIHL with age, sex, rank, duration of service, diabetes and hypertension. These variables were further analyzed by Multiple Logistic Regression and Odds Ratio.

Results

A total of 543 police personnel were identified for the period from January-December 2012. Of this total, 365 were eligible for the study; i.e. there was presence of occupational noise exposure in the shooting range and traffic noise.

The remaining 178 were excluded from study population. Demographic details from this group included 148 (83.1%) male, 30 (16.9%) female, mean age of 36.2 years, mean duration of service 15.8 years. Reasons for their exclusion were: hobbies involving frequent singing or karaoke activities, listening to loud music, part time work in a noisy environment (74, 41.6%): used of ototoxic medications (9, 5.1%): history of head injury (19, 10.7%): family history of hearing loss (19, 10.7%): exposure to solvents (35, 19.7%) and history of chronic ear infection (79, 44.4%).

The descriptive characteristics of the study population and presence
of NIHL are presented in Table 1.

Table 1. Characteristics of study population & presence of NIHL

		Study population (N=365)		Presence of NIHL (n=125)		Excluded population (N=178)
		Mean (SD)	n (%)	Male n (%)	Female n (%)	n (%)
Age (years)		35.55 (9.57)				
Sex	Male		273(74.8)			148(83.1)
	Female		92(25.2)			30(16.9)
Duration of service (years)		14.75 (9.39)				
Presence of NIHL			125(34.2)	103/273 (37.7)	22/92 (23.9)	60(33.7)
Age group (years)	20-29		125(34.2)	11 (10.7)	1 (4.5)	54(30.3)
	30-39		119(32.6)	42 (40.8)	2 (9.1)	60(33.7)
	40-49		79(21.6)	35 (34.0)	7 (31.8)	40(22.5)
	50-59		42(11.5)	15 (14.6)	12 (54.5)	24(13.5)
Duration of service (years)	10-15		206(56.4)	41 (39.8)	1 (4.5)	93(52.2)
	16-30		136(37.2)	52 (50.5)	16 (72.7)	67(37.6)
	31-45		23(6.3)	10 (9.7)	5 (22.7)	18(10.1)
Rank	APO		159(43.6)	21 (16.8)	2(1.6)	70(39.3)
	PC		71(19.5)	32(25.6)	2(1.6)	31(17.4)
	LCPL		56(15.3)	15(12)	6(4.8)	33(18.5)
	CPL		39(10.7)	17(13.6)	6(4.8)	19(10.7)
	SGT		14(3.8)	4(3.2)	3(2.4)	7(3.9)
	S/SGT,SGT/M AJ		16(4.4)	8(6.4)	1(0.8)	7(3.9)
	INSPECT		10(2.7)	6(4.8)	2(1.6)	11(6.2)
Use of ear defenders	Yes		235 (64.4)	64 (62.1)	14 (63.6)	128(71.9)
	No		130 (35.6)	39 (37.9)	8 (36.4)	50(28.1)
Smoking	Yes		162 (44.3)	60 (58.3)	0 (0)	94(52.8)
	No		203 (55.7)	43 (41.7)	22 (100)	84(47.2)
Alcohol consumption	Yes		28 (7.7)	9 (8.7)	1 (4.5)	21(11.8)
	No		337 (92.3)	94 (91.3)	21 (95.5)	157(88.2)
Diabetes Mellitus	Yes		33(9)	13 (12.6)	5 (22.7)	18(10.1)
	No		332(91)	90 (87.4)	17 (77.3)	160(89.9)
Hypertension	Yes		58(15.9)	27 (26.2)	8 (36.4)	29(16.3)
	No		307(84.1)	76 (73.8)	14 (63.6)	149(83.7)
Hyper-cholesterolaemia	Yes		138(37.8)	39 (37.9)	11 (50.0)	52(29.2)
	No		227(62.2)	64 (62.1)	11 (50.0)	126(70.8)

Diabetes mellitus - fasting venous blood glucose level ≥7.0 mmol/L (WHO, 1999).

Hypertension - BP ≥140/90 mm Hg (Willams B, 2004).

Hypercholesterolemia - total fasting cholesterol ≥5.17 mmol/L (NICE, 2008).

The study population was predominantly male (74.8%). The mean age of police personnel was 35.55 years with mean duration of service of 14.75 years. The majority of the personnel (43.3%) were Additional Police Officers (APO) whose job scope included mainly operational duties, whereas the higher ranks handled more administrative duties. 64.4% of the study population used hearing protective devices (ear muffs) during shooting practices whilst 35.6% were non-compliant with this rule. 44.3% were smokers and only 7.7% consumed alcohol.

The results revealed that occupational NIHL was prevalent in 34.2% of police personnel. NIHL was found to be higher in males (37.7%) than in females (23.9%). Males aged 30-39 years (40.8%) and females aged 50-59 years (54.5%) had the highest prevalence rate. Those who served the force for 16 to 30 years recorded the highest prevalence rate for NIHL in both genders (50.5% for males, 72.7% for females). Male personnel in the rank of Police Constable and Additional Police Officer recorded a high prevalence of NIHL (31.1% and 20.4% respectively), whereas in females this was largely seen in the ranks of Lance Corporal (27.3%) and Corporal (27.3%). Interestingly, 62.1% of males with NIHL and 63.6% of females with NIHL used ear muffs during shooting practices. There was a higher percentage of non-diabetics, non-hypertensive and non-hypercholesterolaemics in the NIHL population, with the exception of females in the hypercholesterolemia group where this was seen to be equal (50%).

Table 2. Prevalence of NIHL by degree of severity and gender.

Grade of NIHL[a]		Male n	Female n	Total n (%)
Mild	(26–40 dBA)	43	10	53 (93)
Moderate	(41–60 dBA)	1	1	2 (3.5)
Severe	(61–80 dBA)	2	0	2 (3.5)
Profound	(>80 dBA)	0	0	0 (0)
Total		46	11	57

[a] WHO classification of hearing impairment (WHO, 1991)

Degree of severity of NIHL was further categorized using the World Health Organization (WHO) grading where the average was taken for readings at the lower frequencies 500, 1000, 2000 and 4000 Hertz, in the better impaired ear (WHO, 1991). Out of 125 police personnel with NIHL, 45.6% (57/125) were found to have mild to severe NIHL. Of this, the majority (93%) had mild NIHL, 3.5% had moderate NIHL and another 3.5% had severe NIHL, whilst no police personnel had profound NIHL. There were more males (80.7%) than females who had hearing impairment in the lower frequencies.

Table 3. Factors associated with NIHL.

	OR (95% CI)	X^2(P value)	Multiple Logistic Regression OR (95% CI)	P value
Gender [a]	0.51 (0.30,0.8)	5.8 (0.01)	1.9 (1.1,3.4)	0.01
Age group (years)		63.4 (0.00)	2.5 (1.9,3.2)	0.00
Duration of service (years)		42.3 (0.00)	3.2 (2.2,4.7)	0.00
Rank		60.9 (0.00)	1.5 (1.3,1.7)	0.00
Use of hearing defender [b]	1.14 (0.72,1.78)	0.32 (0.56)		
Smoking [c]	0.80 (0.51,1.23)	1.0 (0.31)		
Alcohol consumption [d]	0.93 (0.41,2.08)	0.29 (0.86)		
Diabetes Mellitus [e]	0.39 (0.19,0.81)	6.63 (0.01)		
Hypertension [f]	0.27 (0.15,0.48)	20.8 (0.00)	3.3 (1.8,6.1)	0.00
Hypercholesterolaemia [g]	0.86 (0.55,1.35)	0.38 (0.53)		

OR – Odds Ratio   CI –Confidence Interval

[a] male (reference group)   [b] uses hearing defender (reference group)

[c] non-smoker (reference group)

[d] does not drink alcohol (reference group)   [e] no Diabetes (reference group)

[f] no Hypertension (reference group) [g] no Hypercholesterolaemia (reference group)

Further analyses showed that some of the factors studied have an association with NIHL

(Table 3). Factors with a strong association are gender, age, duration of service, rank, diabetes mellitus and hypertension. However, only gender and hypertension were strongly associated with NIHL when a multivariate analysis was done, showing that the odds of having NIHL in males was 1.9 times higher than in females, and 3.3 times higher in the hypertensive group.

Discussion

Occupational noise-induced hearing loss is a well-recognized condition amongst police personnel particularly in motorcycle police officers (Shrestha I, et al, 2011). However, only few studies worldwide have been conducted in this occupational group to evaluate associated risk factors. In our study, NIHL was noted to be more prevalent among the male police personnel (37.7%) compared to females (23.9%). This is similar to the findings of other studies [19, 20] where the prevalence of NIHL was found to be 28% in French Police Officers, 66.4% in traffic police personnel in Kathmandu City, 81.2% in Pune traffic police in India and 84% in traffic police in Jalgaon Urban Centre in India. The difference in prevalence may be due to variation in demographic distribution and greater traffic noise pollution in India and Kathmandu than in France. Also, as France is a more developed country, there is better awareness, provision of hearing protective devices and adequate noise conservation programs in place.

Worldwide, 16% of disabling hearing loss in adults is attributed to occupational noise exposure with the effect of exposure being greater in males than females (Nelson DI, et al, 2005). In the United Kingdom, it was estimated that 153,000 men and 26,000 women had severe hearing difficulty were due to occupational noise exposure (Palmer K, et al, 2002). Amongst the United States military personnel, the prevalence of NIHL in males was found to be significantly higher than in females (Helfer TM, et al, 2010).

NIHL was also seen to be more prevalent in the 30-49 years age group in male, as well as in the groups who have served more than

15 years in the police force in Brunei Darussalam. Our result is similar to few other studies which showed that prevalence of NIHL is directly proportional to increasing age and longer duration of service (Masterson EA, et al, 2013).

Our study also showed that the prevalence of NIHL in the group wearing hearing protective devices (ear muffs) was higher than that in the non-hearing defender user group. However, this was not statistically significant and this could be due to improper usage and poor technique when using hearing protective devices. On the other hand, this could also be due to behavioral change for those known to have some hearing impairment resulting in increased use of hearing protective devices in order to prevent further hearing loss. Studies have shown that acute acoustic trauma due to fire arm use in military personnel can be prevented by using appropriate ear defenders which are well fitted for the user during planned training exercises. (Mrena R, et al, 2004).

Some studies have propounded cigarette smoking as an important factor for the increased likelihood of NIHL due to the increased blood viscosity and decreased oxygenation, both of which contribute to impairment of cochlear circulation (Mohammadi S, et al, 2010). In contrast, there are other studies which were not able to show a relationship between smoking and NIHL. Our result is similar to the latter group (Karlsmose B, et al, 2000).

Many studies have looked into the relationship between pre-existing chronic diseases and NIHL, and we attempted to do the same in our local setting in the RBPF. Of the three common chronic diseases studied, only hypertension was found to be statistically significant (p value <0.001). This study showed that those with hypertension were 3.3 times more likely to be associated with NIHL, than those who were non-hypertensive.

Other studies, Talbott E, et al (1985); Toppila E, et al (2000); Johnsson A, et al (1997); and Andren L, et al (1980); have also supported this similar finding. Repeated and prolonged exposure to industrial noise can cause permanent loss of hearing and act as a contributing factor to the rise in blood pressure through a mechanism involving structural adaption of blood vessels. Therefore, noise may be one of several external stimuli contributing to the development of arterial hypertension in man.

WHO estimates that globally 16% of individuals have moderate to greater degree of hearing loss due to occupational noise exposure (Nelson DI, et al, 2005). In our study population, males made up the majority of those found to have NIHL at the lower frequencies. Only few had moderate (3.5%) and severe (3.5%) NIHL, whereas no police personnel had profound NIHL.

Hearing Conservation Program

NIOSH recommends every 3dBA increase in noise level exposure is equivalent to being exposed to double the noise intensity level and therefore should half the amount of time the employee should be exposed to it.

There are different types of controls in order to reduce the risk of excessive noise exposure. As per hierarchy of controls, there are engineering controls, followed by administrative controls and lastly personal protective equipment.

Noise Survey

A hearing conservative program should always begin with a preliminary noise survey. The objective of preliminary noise survey is to identify areas in the work place where workers are exposed to hazardous noise level. The preliminary noise survey should able to provide information on whether a noise problem exists, the extent of the problem and identify areas that should need a detailed noise survey. The detail noise survey obtains information on noise levels at various workstations so as to develop guidelines for engineering and administrative controls. It will also define areas where hearing protection is necessary and identify those employees who would be included in the audiometric testing program (Olishifski and Stanford, 1988).

This program requires employers to monitor noise exposure levels at the worksite in such a way as to identify as accurately as possible the employees who are exposed to noise levels of >85dB averaged per 8 working hours. These employees must be monitored using measurements that are continuous, intermittent and also noise impulses in the 80 – 130dB range. These measurements should be taken in typical working environments. It is also required that employers repeat monitoring in circumstances where production or work process are likely to increase noise exposure for the employees, whom are entitled to observe the monitoring process and it's results.

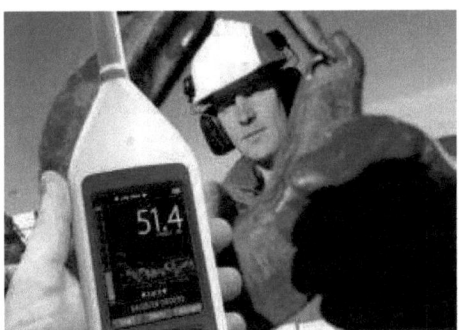

Engineering Controls

Noise control through engineering controls is the most important control measure in a hearing conservative program. Other measures are implemented only when engineering controls are not possible. It is the only method that controls the noise level while other control exposure to noise. Although the initial cost of putting engineering controls in place is high, it must be realized that it is not recurrent expenditure. Complete knowledge is necessary to decide whether noise should be controlled at the source or in the path. Measures of controlling noise at the source include replacing or substituting equipment with less noisy equipment, moving the source further away from the operator, reducing in vibration with vibration absorbing materials or using silencers for air and gas flows. Measures of the noise control in the path include acoustical shields, barrier walls and partial and total closures of the source of noise. In essence, engineering noise control would involve equipment replacement, equipment relocation, vibration isolation, barriers, enclosures, mufflers and source design (Bruce, 1979).

Administrative Controls

When engineering controls are not feasible, administrative controls can be introduced to reduce individual employee exposures. Administrative controls may be implemented by switching employee in high noise area with those in low noise areas after a certain period of time has elapsed. It could also involve scheduling operating time so as to minimize the number of employees exposed to high noise level, for example, ensuring that any noisy equipment are utilised during the time of day when there are least amount of workers at the workplace. Placing a strict limit on the time a worker has to use noisy equipment and all other workers not directly involved with noisy equipment should be placed at a sufficient distance as to reduce exposure to excess noise as much as possible.

Audiometric testing program

Audiometry is not a substitute for noise control. However, an audiometric testing program testing program including baseline, periodic and end of employment audiometry is extremely useful in a hearing conservation program.

Supervision of personnel, approved and calibrated audiometers and approved booths are essentials. Employers must provide baseline audiograms within 6 months of an employee being exposed to working conditions that are about an 8-hour TWA of 85dB. Employees should not be exposed to workplace noise 14 hours prior to the baseline audiogram test. Audiograms should be performed annually thereafter.

Any employee showing standard threshold shift (STS) of 10dB or more @ 2kHz, 3kHz and 4kHz should be provided with adequate hearing protectors, provided for by the employer. If an audiogram shows STS, then the employer is required to notify the employee.

Hearing Protection

Hearing protection is instituted to supplement these control measures. The primary objective in using hearing protectors is to economically reduce hazardous exposure to safely level at the ear of employees to prevent hearing loss. Hearing protectors, e.g; ear plugs, ear muffs and helmets, must be made available to all those exposed to noise levels at or above 85 dBA at no cost to employees. Employees should be able to select the hearing protectors and be provided training in its use and care. Proper fitting of hearing protectors because of the large variation in ear canal diameter and shape is important. Problems are sometimes encountered in finding ear plugs that fit and custom fitted ear plugs may be necessary. The wearing of double protection (for example, ear plugs together with ear muffs) is also strongly recommended especially in working environments exceeding 110 dBA.

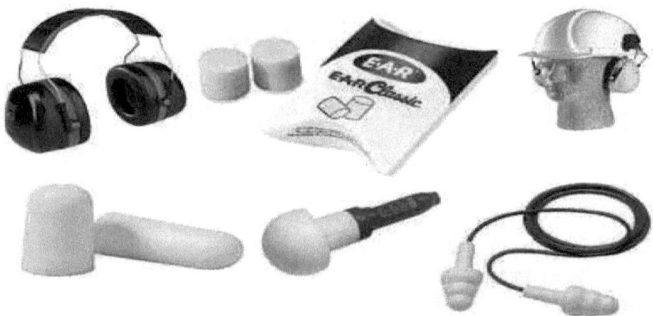

Training and Education

It is vital for the employee to be trained properly of the use of hearing protection and the effects of noise induced hearing loss in order for them to understand the program and be more motivated to wear their protectors and comply with audiometric tests. Training also includes how to properly select the appropriate gear, how the gear should fit and proper are of the hearing protectors. Informing workers of auditory disorders that can occur as a result of noise exposure is important for the success of a hearing conservation program. Employee has a "Right to know" is slowly arriving in developing countries.

Medical Surveillance

Health and Safety Executive (HSE) UK recommends for employees who are at high risk of excessive noise exposure to have a baseline assessment, and then annual medical assessment for two years followed by once every three years (HSE, 2015).

Record Keeping

Employers should keep noise exposure measurement records whilst also maintaining a record of employee's audiogram results for the duration of their contract. A work-related hearing loss register should also be kept by the employer, thereby enabling them to refer to relevant medical professionals if audiograms show a marked decrease in overall hearing. Proper record keeping of exposure and hearing status information is crucial for monitoring and medico-legal purposes. For future medico-legal purposes, records should be kept for at least 30 years (OSHA, 2002).

Potential Pharmacological Treatment of NIHL

The intervention that could reduce damage of hair cell on cochlea by noise that include:

1. Ameliorating lipid peroxidation and cell damages.
2. Ensuring cochlear blood flow during and after noise exposure is not compromised.

Intervention such as antioxidant agents, vasodilator, neurotrophic agents, steroids, calcineurin inhibitors and Src proteintyrosine kinase inhibitors have all been shown to be at least partially effective in preventing hair cell death and subsequent hearing loss (Henderson, et al, 2006). The most effective strategy may include targeting initiating events and maintaining the cell in relatively "normal" physiological state (Le Prell, et al, 2007).

Assessment of Hearing Impairment

Auditory disorders that can affect fitness for work include hearing loss, tinnitus, ear discharge, balance disturbances and problems with barometric pressure differences. While decision on the auditory requirement for fitness for work is usually depend upon specific international regulations and national guidelines of specific country.

Hearing loss can be result from accidents or injuries sustained at work e.g; following blast injury, head injury or barotrauma. The hearing loss may be unilateral or bilateral and it may or may not improved over time. The worker may also be entitled to temporary disability benefits such as medical leave and medical expenses.

The assessment should be carried out when the hearing loss is stabilised and not expected to improve further and it is based on the pure tone audiogram. The audiometric examination should be conducted in proper acoustic environment by trained person. The assessment is based on hearing thresholds for air-conduction. It should be done at least 14 hours noise free period prior to the examination to exclude temporary threshold shift. Comparison should be made with pre-incident or previous audiogram records where these are available. The assessment is always based on better ear and correction should be made for presbycusis for workers who are aged above 50 years (Kumar P, et al, 2006).

The Average Hearing Loss (AHL) of the threshold for 1,2 or 3 kHz is taken and compensation is only payable for hearing loss level of 50 dBa or above (AHL over 1,2, or 3 kHz).

Hearing threshold (dBA) (AHL: 1,2,AND 3 kHz)	Injuries or Accidents (affected ear, % incapacity)	Noise Induced Deafness (better ear, %incapacity)
50	3	5
55	5	10
60	8	15
65	10	20
70	13	25
75	15	30
80	20	40
85	25	50
90	30	60

NB. For sudden hearing loss resulting from accidents or injuries, assess each affected ear and add the percentage incapacities to get the total percentage incapacity. For noise induced hearing deafness, assess the better ear.

Example:

1. A 48 years old worker suffered a sudden hearing loss and tinnitus in both ears after a blast injury at work. He had an AHL (1-3 kHz) of 90 dBA in his left ear and AHL (1-3 kHz) of 60 dBA in his right ear. A prior to the accident, his record showed that his AHL (1-3 kHz) of 40 dBA in his left ear and AHL (1-3 kHz) of 35 dBA in his right ear.

   a. A diagnosis of blast injury of both ears was made.

   b. For the blast injury of left ear, the incapacity was 30%.

   c. The blast injury of the right ear, the incapacity was 8%.

   d. The total incapacity was 30+8 = 38%

2. A 54 years old policeman has been exposed to heavy traffic noise for past 25 years. His audiogram showed bilateral sensorineural hearing loss more pronounced in higher frequencies. His hearing thresholds ranged from 65 to 90 dBA in all frequencies tested. A repeat audiogram showed similar results. His AHL (1-3 kHz) was 75 dBA in the left ear and 60 dBA in Rt ear.

   a. A diagnosis of noise induced deafness (advanced) was made.

   b. The AHL (1-3 kHz) of the better ear was 60 dBA.

c. Based on above table, using column for NID, the percentage is 15%.

d. Correction for prebycusis: minus 2%(4 years above 50)

e. The final incapacity award is 13%.

Limitations of Study

The study team recognize that there were limitations to this study. We were unable to measure the exact level of noise exposure it was not feasible to conduct environmental noise measurement and personal dosimetry at the work place including the shooting range, due to administrative reasons. The Occupational Health Division took over the health surveillance of police personnel in 2005; therefore some of the study subjects who have been in service for long duration may have pre-existing hearing impairment during a time when regular audiometry was not a requirement of their health surveillance hence absence of baseline audiograms.

Conclusion

Diagnosis of NIHL is made when noise exposure is definite and other causes are excluded and it is an incurable but preventable occupational condition. This study shows that increasing age, longer duration of service and presence of hypertension are significant associated factors for NIHL. Preventative strategies such as noise survey, engineering control, administrative control, adequate provision of hearing protective device, regular education and training for employer and employees, implementation of a hearing conservation program (HCP) at the workplace and regular health surveillance (audiometry) for police personnel with exposure to excessive noise, record keeping, can help address the problem.

Our study did not include noise exposure assessment during police shooting practice at the shooting range. Further research could include carrying out field work assessment to identify the exact nature of noise exposure such as impulse or continuous noise, noise levels produced by various types of fire arms and length of exposure time to excessive noise.

References

Andren L, Hansson L, Bjorkman M, Jonsson A. Noise as a contributory factor in the development of elevated arterial blood pressure. Scandinavia Medical Journal 1980; 207: 493-98.

Azizi MH. Occupational Noise-induced Hearing Loss. International Journal Of Occupational and Environmental Medicine. 2010; 1(3).

Birgitta B,Lindvall T, Schwela DH. Guidelines for community noise. World Health Organization Geneva. 1999: 160.

Dobie RA. The burdens of age related and occupational noise induced hearing loss in the United States. 2007; 29(4):545-77.

Fuente A and Hickson L. Noise-induced hearing loss in Asia. International Journal of Audiology 2011; (50)1:S3-10.

Hansen CH. Occupational exposure to noise evaluation, prevention and control; Fundamentals of Acoustic. World Health Organization (Geneva). 1995; 23-51.

Health and Safety Executive (UK) London 2015. *Health surveillance for noise induced hearing loss*, viewed 15 September 2015, http://www.hse.gov.uk/vibration/hav/roadshow/al9.pdf.

Helfer TM, Canham-Chervak M, Canada S, Mitchener TA. Epidemiology of hearing impairment and noise induced hearing loss among US military personnel, 2003-2005. American Journal of Preventive Medicine 2010; 38 (1S): S71-7.

Johnsson A, Hansson L. Prolonged exposure to stressful stimulus (noise) as a cause of raised blood pressure in man. Lancet 1977; 309(8002): 86-87.

Karlsmose B, Lauritzen T, Engberg M, Parving A. A five-year longitudinal study of hearing in a Danish rural population aged 31-50 years. British Journal of Audiology 2000; 34(1): 47-55.

Koh D, Takahashi K; Text book of Occupational Medicine Practice. 3rd ed. Singapore: world Scientific Publishing Co Pte Ltd: January 2011; 310-12.

Kumar P, Chan T C, Sien L K, Chan C, He KK, Siang LH. A Guide to the Assessment of Traumatic Injuries and Occupational Diseases for Workmen's Compensation 5th Edition. Workmen's Compensation Medical Board, Ministry of manpower, Singapore 2006; 66-68.

Le Prell CG, Yamashita D, Minami SB, et al. Mechanism of noise induced hearing loss indicates multiple methods of prevention. Hearing Research Journal Elsevier 2007; 226(1-2):22-43.

Masterson EA, Sang WT, Themann CL, Wall DK, Groenewold MR, Deddens JA, Calvert GM. Prevalence of Hearing Loss in the United States by Industry. American Journal of Industrial Medicine 2013; 56(6): 670-81.

Mc Combe AW, Binnington J, Davis A, Spencer H. Hearing loss and motorcyclists. Journal of Laryngology Otology 1995; 109: 599-604.

Mohammadi S, Mazhari MM, Mehrparvar AH, Attarchi MS. Cigarette smoking and Occupational Noise Induced Hearing Loss. European Journal of Public Health 2010; 20(4): 452-5.

Mrena R, Savolainen S, Pirvola U, Ylikoski J. Characteristics of acute acoustical trauma in the Finnish Defence Forces. International Journal Audiology 2004; 43:177-81.

National Institute for Care Excellence (UK) guideline (reissued March 2010). Cardiovascular risk assessment and modification of blood lipids for the primary and secondary prevention of cardiovascular disease. NICE Guideline (CG 67). May 2008.

Nelson DI, Nelson RY, Concha-Barrientos M, Fingerhut M. The global burden of occupational noise-induced hearing loss. American Journal of Internal Medicine 2005; 48:1-15.

Nelson DI, Robert Y, Marisol CB and Marilyn F. The global burden of occupational noise-induced hearing loss. American Journal of Industrial Medicine 2005 Dec; 48 (6): 446-58

Occupational Safety and Health Administration (OSHA). Hearing Conservation. OSHA, US Department of Labour. Washington, OSHA 3074; 2002:1-8.

Palmer K, Griffin M, Sydall HE, Davis A, Pannett B, Coggon D. Occupational exposure to noise and attributable burden of hearing difficulties in Great Britain. Occupational Environmental Medicine 2002; 59(9): 634-9.

Ross BC. Noise exposure of motorcyclists. Annals of Occupational Hygiene 1989; 33: 123-7.

Samant Y, Parker D, Wergeland E, Wannag A. The Norwegian Labour Inspectorate's Registry for Work-Related Diseases: data from 2006. Journal of Occupational and Environmental Health 2008; 14(4): 272-79.

Shrestha I, Shrestha BL, Polharel M, Amatya RCM, Karki DR. The Prevalence of Noise Induced Hearing Loss among Traffic Police Personnel of Kathmandu Metropolitan City. Kathmandu University Medical Journal 2011; 36(4): 274-8.

Steve C, Gunn P, Susan L, Liz W, Cassandra G, Adeline O, Rob M. Safe work. Occupational Noise Induced Hearing Loss in Australia 2010:11-12.

Talbott E, Helmkamp J, Mathews K, Kuller L, Cottington E, Redmond G. Occupational Noise Exposure, Noise Induced Hearing Loss and Epidemiology of High Blood Pressure. American Journal of Epidemiology 1985; 121(4): 501-14.

Toppila E, Pyykko I, Starck J, Kaksonen R, Ishizaki H. Individual risk factors in the development of noise induced hearing loss. Noise & Health 2000; 2(8): 59-70.

Vallet M & Vernet I. Night aircraft noise index and sleep research results. In A. Lawrence (ed.), Inter-Noise 91. The cost of Noise. Noise Control Foundation. New York 1991;(1):207-10.

Willams B, Poulter NR, Brown MJ, Davis M, McInnes GT, Potter JF, Sever PS, Thom MS. British Hypertension Society guideline for hypertension management 2004. British Medical Journal 2004; 328(7440): 634-40.

World Health Organization, Geneva (1991). Report of the Informal Working Group on Prevention of Deafness and Hearing Impairment, Programme Planning. 18-21 June 1991; WHO/PDH/91.1

World Health Organization, Geneva. *Definition, Diagnosis and Classification of Diabetes Mellitus and its Complication 1999.* http://www.who.int/iris/handle/10665/66040#sthash.kAYOLBXT.dp uf

World Health Organization Geneva. *Prevention of blindness and deafness. Facts about Deafness 2012,* viewed on 15 November 2013, http://www.who.int/pbd/deafness/facts/en/.

Principal Author – Dr Kyaw Naing Win

Co- Author – Dr Rizal Sablee

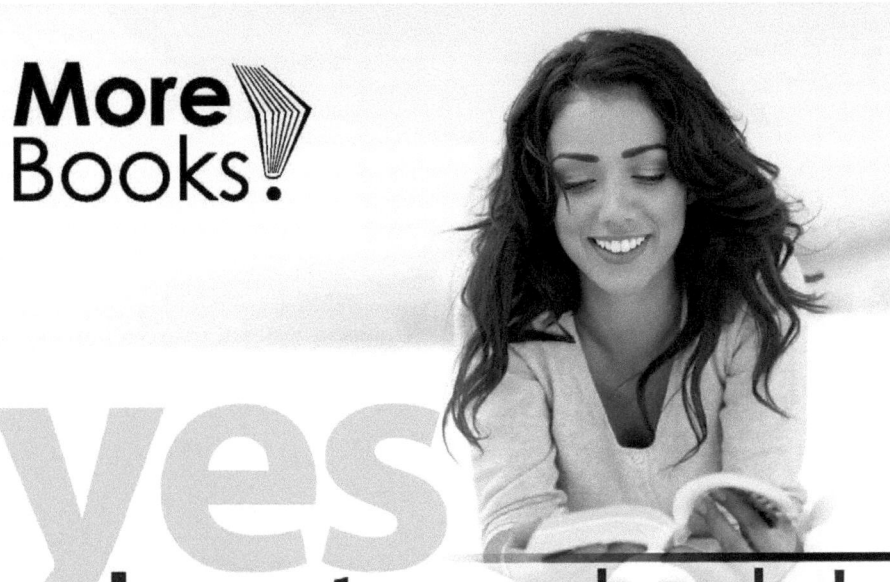
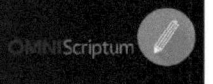

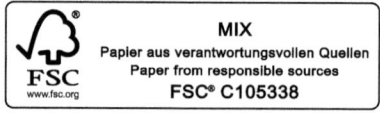